CARE AND FEEDING OF THE LONG WHITE CANE:

Instructions in
Cane Travel
for Blind People

by Thomas Bickford

D1382638

Large Type Edition

published by
NATIONAL FEDERATION OF THE BLIND

TABLE OF CONTENTS

Thoughts and Experiences on Cane Travel

Songs

ACKNOWLEDGEMENTS

Virginia, Ann, and Barbara—my wife and daughters—make my life and work worthwhile and possible. Here are my love and support.

Dr. Kenneth Jernigan has for me, as for so many others, been my mentor and guide. He taught me what I know about blindness and showed me that I could live a full life. He also gave me comments on this booklet.

For their support, inspiration, and comments, I thank my friends in the National Federation of the Blind: Lloyd Rasmussen, Judy Rasmussen, Debbie Brown, Arlene Hill, Sharon Duffy, and Mary Ellen Gabias.

Any writer needs to find and gain access to relevant material, and I was helped by Norma Belt, my reader, and Carol Strauss, reference librarian.

I appreciate the discussions of shared experiences with Alan and Billie Ruth Schlank. As a beginning author, I appreciate the help in editing offered by Carl Knoettner. I thank my students who taught me as I was teaching them.

WHY LARGE TYPE

The type size used in this book is 14 Point for two important reasons: One, because typesetting of 14 Point or larger complies with federal standards for the printing of materials for visually impaired readers, and we wanted to show you exactly what type size is necessary for people with limited sight.

The second reason is because many of our friends and supporters have asked us to print our paperback books in 14 Point type so they too can easily read them. Many people with limited sight do not use Braille. We hope that by printing this book in a larger type than customary, many more people will be able to benefit from it.

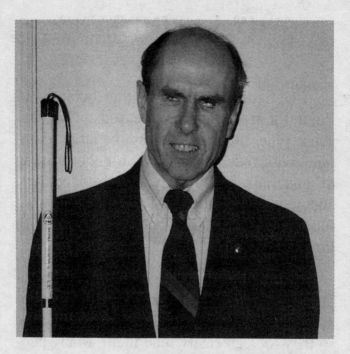

Tom Bickford

ABOUT THE AUTHOR

Thomas Bickford became blind at the age of seventeen from glaucoma. Mr. Bickford started using a cane during the summer between high school and college because his sight was fading past the point of usefulness for travel. He learned some basic cane techniques from a fellow college student. After college, he attended the California Orientation Center for the Blind where, among other things, he took formal instruction in cane travel and met and joined the National Federation of the Blind. Mr. Bickford holds his B.A. degree from Occidental College, Los Angeles, and his M.A. degree from the University of Iowa, Iowa City. For the past twenty-six years Mr. Bickford has worked for the Library of Congress, National Library Service for the Blind and Physically Handicapped in Washington, D.C. He makes his home in suburban Maryland with his wife and two daughters. Since people ask how much a blind traveler can see, Mr. Bickford speaks of himself as "very totally blind."

To L. Q. "Larry" Lewis.

May he rest in peace because I walk with confidence.

AUTHOR'S INTRODUCTION

This booklet contains the experience and observations I have gained over many years as a cane traveler. My hope is to share these experiences and observations with you. But the booklet cannot go with you to say, "You are doing that right, but you need to do it twenty-five or thirty times, not just two or three times." It cannot say, "Swing your cane farther to the left, but not quite so far to the right." The booklet cannot follow you around the block to say, "Yes, this block really does have four corners, but you were off course when you went around one of the corners, and you didn't recognize it." The booklet cannot tell you at which moment it is safe to cross a street, nor should it try to tell you where particular obstacles are. To become an independent traveler you must, and I believe you can, learn to take care of yourself. The best thing this booklet can do for you is to help you come to the time when you don't need it.

A skilled and knowledgeable teacher might help you learn that combination of skills that make up cane travel, and the process might go faster. Such a teacher could present new challenges at the right time or help review persistent problems. I think of this part of the process as "guided practice," and it was very helpful to me. If you had such a teacher, you might not be reading this booklet, so let's get on with the process.

"In avoiding the discomfort of fearful feelings you also eliminate the opportunity for courageous actions, ... and the emotional maturity such action develops. If you happen to feel fear, and who doesn't, don't duck it; use it."

—Nancy Mairs. *Carnal Acts*. New York: Harper Collins, 1991.

"We should use technology only where it's necessary. Throughout my career in this field there have been flurries of interest in mobility devices, and I've always felt that the ordinary cane, which is technologically simple, is, in fact, very sophisticated and sufficient for the job."

—Raymond Kurzweil. Technology Producers Present Their Views: The First Panel, Remarks by Raymond Kurzweil. *The Braille Monitor*, January, 1992, p. 22.

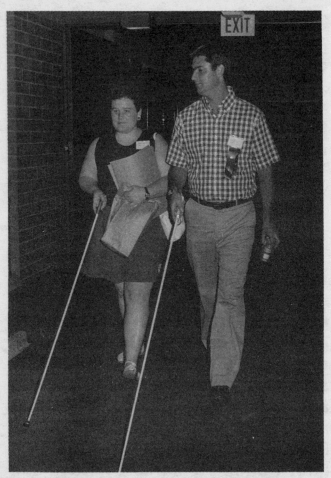

People who use canes well travel rapidly and efficiently.

■ GETTING YOURSELF READY

Why Should I Use This Thing That Makes Me Look Blind?

One of the reasons that makes me qualified to ask this question and offer an answer is that I asked myself this same question when I got my first cane. When I asked the lady who sold me the cane in the local agency for the blind, "How do I use it?" her answer was, "Any way you like."

I was in my last year of high school then, losing sight slowly but steadily, and we all know how high school students hate to look "different." As I walked with my parents across the street back to the car, I pondered the more basic question, "Why use this cane at all?"

Through the National Federation of the Blind I learned that there are two major schools of thought about what it means to be blind. One philosophy of blindness held by most people, including many blind people, says that blindness is a disaster, a catastrophe. I tell you frankly and up front, if you decide that blindness is a disaster, it will be for you. It will dominate and ruin your life. It will limit your thoughts, your relationships and your achievements.

The NFB taught me the other philosophy of blindness, that blindness is a physical characteristic, that with the right approach and with the right kinds of training in dealing with the situations you meet in your daily life, blindness can be reduced to a matter of nuisance value. Some nuisances are bigger than others, but blindness no longer has the power to dominate and ruin your life. But this learning was a few years in the future, so back to my late teens.

I don't know anyone who wants to be blind. I hated to admit that I was blind, because it was a change in my self-image. I still had that majority view of blindness, that it was a terrible thing. I knew that the white cane identified me as a blind person, and I only thought of this negative purpose.

The cane has a functional purpose, and that is what most of the rest of this booklet is about. I started carrying the cane because I was losing more sight and running into too many things. I just held it out in front of me with an occasional swing to the side to check for landmarks. A few months later I met a blind veteran who used a long cane and had good travel skills. He taught me enough to keep me going in limited situations.

Another way to think of the cane is as a magic wand. If you know anything about magic tricks, you know that the magician must practice for hours before going on stage for a performance. The magic tricks that you perform with the cane, threading your way past obstacles and finding your destination, come with hours of practice. I will tell you how long it took me to learn, and it was well worth the time and effort. Now to return to the question of looking like a blind person.

The better I grew as a cane traveler, the less it bothered me to carry a cane. The better I grew as a cane traveler, the less people asked if I wanted help. The better I grew as a cane traveler, the less it bothered me when people did offer help. I knew where I was going, and it showed. I looked like a capable person. A skillful blind traveler draws attention in the same way that a beautiful woman or handsome man draws attention. People notice, admire for a moment, and then go on their way as you go on yours. But I would have found all that hard to believe at the beginning.

There are times when it is appropriate for people to know that I am blind. The cane is a silent explanation when I enter a bank and ask where the end of the teller's line is. I give all my attention to traffic when I cross streets, but I want the driver approaching the corner to know that I am blind. I try not to "wave the white cane" when I could do things for myself, because that works against opening opportunities for achievement in other areas of my life. But that is another chapter in the philosophy of blindness.

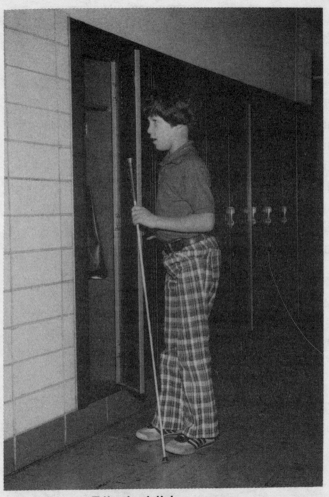

*Blind children use
their canes in school.*

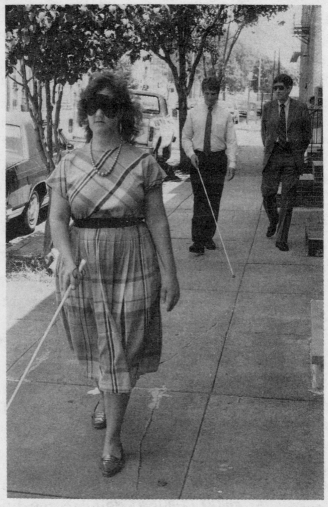

Cane techniques are easily learned.

Who Can Learn Cane Travel?

Let's turn away from cane travel for a moment and consider swimming. To a non-swimmer or even an impartial observer who is standing on the ground, the idea of swimming is foolish. They might say, "Humans can't do that. We don't have air sacs along our spines like fish. Our only air sacs expand and contract with every breath."

Have you ever seen or been a non-swimmer in the water, the way they thrash around? "Water is too thin. It will not support you, and you will soon drown." Even if the observer sees someone else swimming, the response is, "Maybe they can do it, but I couldn't. And who would want to do that, anyway? I can go all the places I want to go my own way."

The only way to learn to swim is to actually get into the water. Yes, at first you do thrash around, and sink, and come up coughing with your eyes and nose full of water. It takes a while to learn how to relax the right way to let the water support you. Much of the skill in swimming is in learning to cooperate with the water and to use its properties to help you do what you want to do.

In every society there are skills that people are expected to learn and to perform well. Up until a hundred years ago Native American men and boys were expected to be skillful in the use of the bow and arrow. Allowing for individual variations, I am sure that most of them were skillful.

Since everyone eats, lots of people need to cook, and cooking is a skill that many people can learn to a satisfactory degree. There is another factor involved in cooking, just as there was in the use of the bow and arrow: separation by gender. Women were not expected to shoot the bow and arrow, and, even now, many men are not expected to cook.

Early in my career I worked in a recreation center. Near closing time one day I remarked to one of the boys that I had to go home and cook my dinner. To him, that was a ridiculously funny idea, and all he could say was, "Cooking is women's work!" It was no good telling him that I lived alone and had no one to cook for me. This time, at least, it had nothing to do with my blindness.

There is one thing that all American adults are expected to do, and that is to drive a car. There are a few parallels between any two forms of transportation: noticing surroundings, keeping track of turns and distances, and planning your destination and route. Everyone is expected to do these things. They are basically the same if you are going from one room to another, or from one city to another. The necessary skills are within everyone's range of abilities. I base my opinion on the fact that so many blind people do travel successfully. It takes training and practice, but that is to be expected.

People who can see are used to looking at everything they do, and so they think they have to look in order to know and to do anything. The National Federation of the Blind is in the process of teaching people that it is not so. We expect blind people to learn how to do many things. We lead by example, and offer help along the way. "Here is a cane. Tap it back and forth in front of you as you walk." The cane, itself, is a simple thing. As you step "most of what you need to know is in your head, and that is as good as it ever was."

There is one essential thing that the student must bring to cane travel, and that is the willingness to try. Are there doubts? I had many doubts. Are there fears? I had my share of fears. Is there confusion? I had handfuls of confusion. Are there questions? I had a list of questions which I asked at the wrong times. But along with my doubts, fears, confusions and questions I brought a willingness to try. Many times I repeated lessons, but I kept trying. If you have come this far in the booklet, you can make it the rest of the way. From here on, you need take only a small step at a time, so give it a try.

◼ GETTING THE CANE READY

How Long Should the Cane Be?

I have slowly graduated from a cane that was 42 inches long to a cane that is over 60 inches long. I added a few inches every few years when I bought a new cane. I have not yet had a cane that was too long. My chin-high cane is barely long enough for me now. There are blind people who use canes that reach their eyebrows.

Once while I was teaching travel, it occurred to me that what mattered was not where the cane came on your body, but where it reached in front of you. The speed of your pace and the length of your stride will make a difference. The cane needs to reach a good two steps in front of where you are stepping. As a practical matter, if you find yourself overstepping the cane, dropping off curbs you didn't find, try a longer cane.

When you select a cane, start with one that comes into your armpit. Walk up to a blank wall, swinging the cane from side to side two inches wider than the width of your shoulders. As you step left, tap right; as you step right, tap left. When the cane hits the wall, complete the step you are making, and take one more. Was there space for that next step? If so, you have enough stopping distance. If not, add another two or four inches to the cane and try again. I am not the only one who needs the length of that second step for stopping distance.

Remember that not all obstacles are found at the distance of the end of the cane. You find some things as the cane swings to the side after the tip has passed them. If part of the obstacle is above ground level, such as a chair or a car, part of the cane will pass under it before making contact, and you will be glad to have the added length. You may think that the longer the cane, the more it will get tangled up in whatever is ahead of you, but that can happen with any length of cane.

There is one other factor that I must consider for my cane: will it fit in the family car? The answer is: "Yes, but I have to work at it a bit." The way that is best for me is to bring the handle end in first and push it back as far as possible between the seat and the side of the car. I try to get it under the seat belt anchor and as low as possible, where it won't trip back seat passengers going in and out. The last thing is to make sure the tip end is in the car and not sticking out between the door and the frame. I am not the only person to destroy a cane that way. I am afraid I have made the process sound harder than it is. A couple of pushes and a pull get the cane in position, and it takes less time than fastening a seat belt.

What Should the Cane Be Made Of?

I have used canes made of wood, aluminum tubing, solid fiberglass, fiberglass tubing, and carbon fiber compound tubing. Each material has different characteristics of strength, weight, and flexibility. Each one sounds different as it strikes the ground. I have not used wooden canes or canes with curved handles since the 1950's. White support canes are available for people who need a cane to lean on.

Aluminum tubing canes are relatively heavy and strong. They do not break. If they are bent a little, they will straighten out. With a little more pressure, they will stay bent; very few people have the coordinated strength to return aluminum canes to their original condition. Slightly bent canes may not look as pretty as straight ones, but you can use them for a long time.

Solid fiberglass canes (called rigid because they have no joints) are both strong and flexible, and I like that combination of qualities. They weigh less than aluminum canes, and more than the next two hollow canes. Solid fiberglass will take quite a bend and still straighten. If they are bent past a certain point, they will split into long splinters which are dangerous to touch. The cane will probably get you home in that condition, but beware the splinters.

Hollow fiberglass is lightweight and very easy to handle. It has a nice bounce to it, but will only take a moderate bend without breaking. That is, it may not withstand tripping someone. When it breaks, hollow fiberglass tends to crush and fall apart very soon.

Carbon fiber canes are fairly stiff and have only a little bounce. They are light weight and easy to handle. Compared to hollow fiberglass, the carbon fiber cane is somewhat stronger and lasts a little longer after a break.

I do not know any cane that will withstand being caught in a car door unscathed. I keep a spare cane at home.

Let us consider folding canes. Do not let yourself fall into the trap of thinking you are hiding your blindness by using a folding cane. Also, for at least the duration of the learning stage, I strongly recommend a one-piece cane. There are many blind people who use a folding cane all the time and find it fully satisfactory. For several years I was one of them. The previous section on the length of the cane should still be considered. I often take my folding cane to church, restaurants, theaters—places where it may not be as convenient to stow the one-piece cane.

Many folding canes are made of aluminum tubing sections with some kind of elastic in the middle to pull the sections together. Each producer has his own variation on the way the sections join, so you must make your own choice. Some canes are made of concentric tubing that collapses each one into the next. If you pull each section out firmly and give it a slight twist, it should stay in position during your trip. Both fiberglass and carbon fiber compound are available in this telescoping style.

How and Where Do You Hold the Cane?

The handle goes diagonally across my palm and rests on the extended index finger. The other fingers curl around, and the thumb points over the handle and down the cane. The palm is vertical as when extended to shake hands. That is the classic grip which I use most of the time. In close quarters I slide my hand down the cane and narrow the swing. I may shift my grip and hold the cane like a long pencil. You can't swing the cane much in that position, but you don't want to swing it much because of the crowd. In very close, slow-moving crowds such as in theater lobbies or a line to board a bus, I may just hold the cane diagonally across my body and slide the cane along in front of my left foot. At other times I may shift my grip to ease fatigue or for no special reason.

The firmness of the grip should be moderate, neither so tight that you never let go—

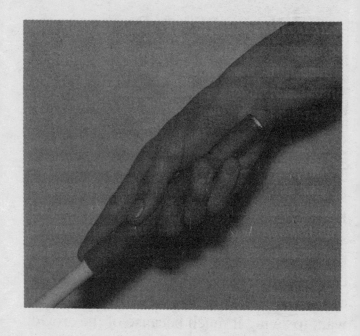

It's important to learn to hold the cane correctly.

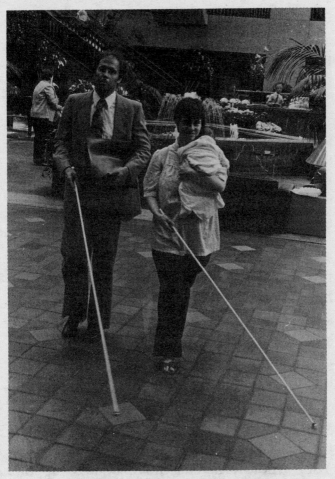

*A properly arcing cane assures
the user that the path is clear.*

you'll break the cane when it gets caught in a crack—nor so loose that every obstacle knocks it out of your hand—you'll have to chase it too often.

I swing the cane from side to side with pressure of the wrist and fingers. The hand swings like a door with the hinge at the wrist. Pretty soon you will be almost flipping the cane back and forth with an easy, unconscious motion.

My first teacher told us to hold the cane just below the belt buckle with the forearm braced against the hip. From that central position the cane can be tapped evenly from side to side. This position is good for beginners, and some people stay with it. Over the years my cane hand has drifted to the side by my pocket. In either position, hold your hand out a few inches so you do not impale yourself when the cane hits a stop. Your whole arm can move to take up the shock.

When you are standing still, hold the cane vertically near your body with a light grip. That is, I don't think you want to look like a shepherd leaning on his staff.

There will be times, walking or standing, when you want to reach out and check a particular landmark or shoreline. Be sure you are not going to trip someone with the sudden motion, reach out, and then bring your arm back to the original position. The point is that you should hold the cane in a manner and position so as to reach where you need to with comfort and without undue fatigue.

Many canes have a loop of chain or string through the handle which is for the purpose of hanging up the cane when it is not in use. Do not put your hand through the loop when you are walking. If something should happen to pull the cane out of your hand, it is better to drop the cane than to be pulled down with it.

You may think I don't care how you hold your cane. I do think that there is more than one way and more than one place to hold the cane. However and wherever you hold the cane, give yourself protection for the full width of your body. The purpose of the grip and position is to make it possible to tap the cane from side to side, which is the subject of the next section, and that is very important.

■ ACTUALLY WALKING AROUND

Walking with the Cane, <u>Rule One</u>

My first travel teacher taught us <u>Rule One</u>: "When the body is in motion, the cane is in rhythm." That means: tap the cane from side to side, one tap per step, about two inches beyond the width of your shoulders. Keep the tip low, but not constantly dragging on the ground.

The idea of Rule One is to clear an area, and step into it. Clear the next area, and step into it. You can do it faster than you can say it. As you step left, tap right; as you step right, tap left. As a beginner, you may think that swinging the cane beyond your shoulders is too wide, but you will learn soon enough that you need the width. With the right length of cane and using this technique, you can learn to walk safely and with confidence. You will locate obstacles and drop-offs and be prepared for them. If you keep the taps at a steady two inches beyond your shoulders, it will help to even out your stride and keep you walking straight. In crowds or other close quarters, shorten up on the handle and narrow your swing. You are still a member of the human race, so remember your basic courtesies.

The cane, of course, will not find every small obstacle on the ground. It can go around an obstacle the size of a brick, but it will find things larger than that. Sometimes there are holes in the sidewalk, and the cane may go completely over a dip the size of a dinner plate or a place mat. True, the cane is not perfect, but nothing else is, either. Sighted or blind, all have stories of how they tripped over or stepped into something.

The cane can tell you what is ahead, but be sure to give it the chance to do that. If you are about to turn in an open area or go around a corner, let the cane clear the area before you step there. The headlights on a car point straight ahead and do not look around the corner before the car turns. With a cane you can and should check the area where you are about to turn and step; side-stepping can be dangerous.

There are many unnumbered lesser rules, but always remember Rule One: "When the body is in motion, the cane is in rhythm."

Planning Practice Routes

In the beginning a straight route is suitable. Try walking up and down your block a time or two while concentrating on <u>Rule One</u>. As you walk you may find a "shoreline" on one side: a wall, a fence, or grass. Let your cane touch the shoreline each time the swing goes to that side. It can help to keep you on course. Shorelines have breaks and irregularities which soon become landmarks to help you keep track of where you are. Soon you will be walking around the block, if your neighborhood is laid out that way, and returning to the starting point. You will find both fixed and movable obstacles, all part of cane travel.

How can you match your next challenge to your level of experience? You may just go a little farther every day. Guided practice can be helpful if you can get it, but I mentioned that at the beginning, so I will not belabor the point.

Going Up and Down Stairs

You're not going to be a flatlander for the rest of your life. Almost every building has stairs or steps somewhere.

You are at the bottom of the stairs, about to go up. Some stairs have handrails, and some don't, and you need to be able to use either kind. If you are using the handrail, put your cane in the other hand. Either way, the cane can tell you how high and deep the first step is. I slide my hand part-way down the cane and hold it diagonally across my body. The cane taps two or three steps ahead of my feet. Going up and down stairs is almost the only place I will tell you not to swing the cane from side to side. At the top, resume <u>Rule One</u>.

When going down, locate the top step first with the cane, then with the foot. Whether or not you use the handrail, hold the cane diagonally across your body. Let the cane tip slide off each step as you go. At the bottom, resume <u>Rule One</u>. There are complications such as landings with or without turns. No one can list all the tricks that architects can imagine. Let your cane go first, and pay attention to what it says.

After this, you will be going up and down the ordinary hills and valleys of the outdoor world.

Listening to Traffic on the Street as a Guide

Cars are a common part of the world we live in. Cars usually drive straight along streets and turn at corners. Yes, I know ... but there are crazy blind pedestrians just as there are crazy sighted drivers.

I have found that a steady stream of traffic is one of the best helps there is. By listening to traffic I can tell how far away

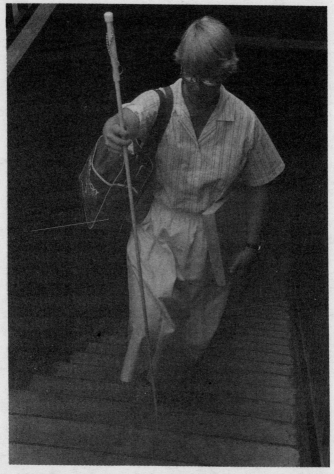

Holding the cane properly is important for going up and down steps.

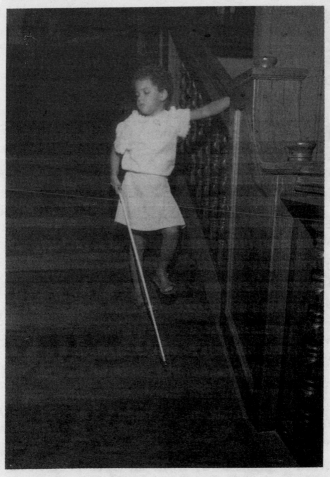

*Even children can use the cane
reliably on the stairs.*

the street is, if the street runs straight or turns, where the intersection is, and which color is showing on the traffic light. I use traffic as an audible shoreline.

When you are walking around the block for practice, I recommend that you do not turn the corner when you think you are there. Go all the way to the curb, then back up a few steps and turn. It is easy for beginners to turn too soon and find themselves without the expected landmarks. Now that you have learned about walking straight and listening to traffic, let's go on to crossing streets.

Crossing Streets with No Traffic

For purposes of practice, use a street with as little traffic as possible. Because many corners are rounded off for the convenience of turning traffic, you cannot just walk straight away from the curb. You need to find something as a guide to be sure you are starting off straight across the street. That guide may be part of the curb beyond

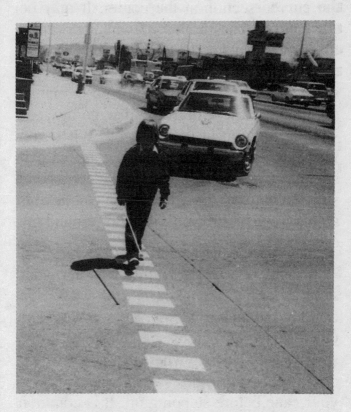

Crossing streets is easy for those who know how to listen.

the curved section at the corner. It may be the dividing lines in the sidewalk. It may be the curb ramp for wheelchairs, but be sure that the ramp is aimed directly across the street and not diagonally out into the intersection. It may be traffic either going your way or crossing in front of you. When you locate your guide, line yourself up with it so that you are facing directly across the street. Listen carefully to be sure that no cars are approaching from the side or around the corner.

Having checked your direction and your safety, step off the curb and walk. Go quickly without rushing. Remember <u>Rule One</u>. There can be obstacles or holes in the street as well as anywhere else. When you come to the far side, sweep the curb with your cane before stepping up. It is common to find signposts near intersections, and I have found some with my head because I didn't find them with my cane. Did you cross straight and arrive at the sidewalk? If not, and I don't always myself, pause to make an educated guess from your surroundings, and make the necessary corrections. There you are across the street. Now you can go on your way.

Which Way Can Cars Turn
At Intersections?

When you consider intersections, you need to know the directions and paths that cars take when they go through or turn. That is: if you are facing a street with the intersecting street on your right, and each street allows two-way traffic, a left-turning car can go from the middle lane on your right to the middle lane in front of you. If you are crossing then, the car will appear to approach from behind your right shoulder. If your experience does not include such information, it is time to learn. You can either observe for yourself or ask for help. There are many combinations of factors to know about including one-way streets, right turn on red, special turning lanes, traffic islands, and traffic lights to accommodate all of these. All drivers out there have to learn the rules of traffic, and you are just as smart as they are. Learn them one at a time as you find them.

Environmental Clues and Mental Maps

In some ways, this section is the heart of cane travel. By using your cane, which I do, or a little sight, which I do not do, you are only extending the range of your perception a few feet. By listening to the sounds around you and the nature of those sounds, you are extending the range of your perception for many feet, sometimes hundreds of feet. The mind has the greatest reach, and can consider distances from inches away to miles away, and objects the size of a bump in the sidewalk to a sports stadium. The mind can form a mental picture or map arranging landmarks along in the right order. Then it can check off each point as you pass it. The mind coordinates all your knowledge, information, senses and skills, so let us use this marvelous mind of ours.

<u>Rule One</u> says: "When the body is in motion, the cane is in rhythm." The cane is good at gathering short-range information for you to act on. The mind needs to be aware of the messages that the cane is sending. The cane sends such messages as: the next step is clear, stop, jog to the side, make a sharp turn, step up or down.

I am sure you have heard someone talking who, in the middle of a sentence, turned his head or put his hand over his mouth. You noticed the change in the character of the sound. The same kind of change happens when the speaker walks around a corner. We can learn to hear these same changes outside while we are walking.

When I became blind, I began to listen to sounds more carefully. Even when I was told about some sounds, I did not notice them. I learned gradually, not all at once. For me, "gradually" meant from a few weeks to a few years.

I found that the sound of a car driving down the street changed when it passed by a parked car or a tree. The first time I remember noticing that effect was when I was still sighted, but temporarily blind. That is, I walked between two parked cars in a <u>very</u> dark parking lot and "heard" them, even though they were standing still. What I heard was the sound shadow, the difference in the background sound as these large objects blocked part of what I heard. It makes no difference what you call this effect, but it may help you if you use the experience. Sometimes you can identify or locate an object by noticing the air currents moving around it, be it a natural breeze or one caused by human action.

When you walk down a hall in a large building, you sometimes pass a door with noise coming out of it. You may approach the intersection of another hall where people are passing by in front of you. The time may come when you notice the open door or the intersecting hall just by the nature of the background sound.

There are more than the five senses of touch, taste, smell, sight, and hearing. There is the sense in our muscles that tells us where our various body parts are. There are also the senses of time and distance. These two work together and can be put to use keeping track of where we are.

At home and work, I know about how big the rooms are and how long the halls are, so I get used to how long it takes to cross a room or to get to the end of the hall. Having gone far enough, I anticipate the next thing to do, which is usually to turn a corner or enter a doorway. When walking outside, we make use of the same senses. We just expand the distances.

One more of the senses is the sense of turning. This sense is not exact to me. I can identify turns better when I am going fast than when I am going slow. Sometimes I walk around a gentle curve and do not know how much I have turned, or that I have turned at all. I wish I could do better.

Once, just for practice, a friend and I stood between a table and a wall and tried to turn exactly 90 degrees back and forth. It helped somewhat. This sense, alone, is not reliable to me, but it is a help when combined with the other senses.

As a new travel student, I asked my teacher, "How can I go two or three blocks this way, and four or five blocks that way, and find the barber shop?" I learned later how much of a "beginner's question" that was. It is like the algebra student who comes to the first class and opens the book in the middle, only to ask, "How can I ever solve that problem?" The answer is that you start at the beginning, and later, when you pass that point in the book you find that it was just one more step along the way. Long ago I found that I could make use of general directions, and I did find the barber shop.

I can usually keep track of where I am by checking off local landmarks and noticing distances, but sometimes I do get confused, disoriented, or simply "lost." I ask directions or pick out a particular spot and do some limited exploring. I may have been a block short, 90 degrees off course, or even right on course but not aware of it. I may feel stupid for a minute, but I get "found" and go on my way.

I learn easily from spacial displays. I like two-dimensional paper maps, but they are hard to find.

When I think of where I'm going, I map out my route in my head. For some people, maps are of no help at all. They do not want to know north and south. Just tell them left or right, and how far it is. I can work from either kind of directions. We all have different abilities, notice different landmarks, and go on different trips, so use the things that help you.

Compass directions can be a very useful tool. First, you need to know that north and south are opposite each other, and that east and west are opposite each other. When you face north, west is to the left and east is to the right. Many cities try to have some orientation to the compass, but there are usually a few streets that curve or are just not straight with the compass. When walking inside a large building, it may be helpful to identify halls by compass directions.

Let me end this section with a set of directions I once gave to a friend of mine. "Go out of the building and turn left to the corner. Cross the street to the right and go south, down to the next corner. You need to cross the intersection both ways, and end up going left, east, for two blocks. That is where you come to the big, wide street with the traffic island on the far side and the separate light for the small street beyond it. When you get across there, turn right, and you will be going slightly downhill. A little way down the block, the street makes a slight turn to the left. From that point on, there are several store entrances that are similar. The one you want is the fourth or fifth one, but it is the only one with a rubber doormat." He said he went right to it.

Expanding Your Horizons

If you are starting cane travel without formal training, you will meet these conditions in no special order. You can learn them as you come to them.

An experienced guide or teacher can be of help in judging the degree of your ability so as to present new challenges at the right time with the right degree of complication. Do you need more practice going around the block so you don't get confused crossing the alley? Do you still pass that store that is set back from the street? Are you keeping track of the landmarks along the route so you know when to turn into the office you wanted to find? On a round trip, can you get back to your starting point?

Landmarks can be such things as a particular arrangement of signposts, mailboxes, lawns, bushes, driveways, barking dogs, busy streets, broken sidewalks, hot-dog stands and gas stations. I have deliberately mentioned things that you feel with a cane, feel with your feet, hear or smell. All of these things have, at times, been landmarks for me. Every blind traveler will develop his own local list of landmarks.

Do you need to take a route down a narrow sidewalk with parking meters every ten feet? That will help you learn how wide to swing your cane and how to get it untangled from obstacles. Do you need to take a route along a very wide sidewalk with crowds of people going both ways, or no other people going either way? That will help you develop your ability to walk straight.

By the way, what is "walking straight?" It is a matter of keeping the goal ahead of you and making a series of minor course corrections. As you gain experience in swinging your cane evenly, as you pick up a little bit of speed, as you make use of more landmarks, and as you identify more sounds around you, you will find that you are walking straight. I listen in all directions, but we usually walk in the direction we are looking, so keep your face straight ahead.

Every now and then someone calls to me, usually from at least 20 feet away, while I am crossing a street, "Straighten out, you're walking crooked!" Of course, had I known I was walking crooked, I would already have made my own corrections. It finally occurred to me that what these people are trying to say is, "You are going off at an angle to the desired direction, and it would be well to alter your course slightly." The person has an idea of what the ideal course would be, but they did not tell me which way to go, left or right. At times like that, I make a quick decision based on what is around me. Oh, when will people learn to be more specific and do it without informing the whole neighborhood?

As I walk down a block in either a business or residential area, I listen to what is around me and what is ahead of me. What is ahead soon becomes the next intersection. By the time I arrive I usually know what the traffic condition is and which street has the green light. If you can learn to add this trick to your list, it will keep you going more smoothly.

One Dangerous Situation to Avoid

Let me tell you of one time <u>not</u> to cross a street. When a car that could go past stops, and the driver calls to you, "Go ahead, I'll wait for you," and especially if there is an empty lane beside the car, <u>do not cross</u>. The time will come when a second driver will not see you and will zip past at speed. Why not? The lights will be with him. I have narrowly escaped injury in such a situation. I went to the funeral of a couple who were caught in just such a situation. Having learned my lesson, I sometimes have to turn and walk away from the curb a few steps in order to convince the driver that I will not cross then.

Crossing Big, Busy Intersections

Busy intersections usually have traffic lights with lots of cars going through. I use the sound of the traffic to show where, when, and how far I need to go. Consider the possibility of such things as traffic islands and multiple phases in the traffic lights. With as much traffic as there is, you could line up your shoulders parallel with the cars crossing in front of you or find some mark on the sidewalk to point you straight across the street. Do not start partway through a cycle on a "stale green" light. I am always wary of people who tell me, "You can go now. There's no one coming." Where I live, drivers observe traffic lights more strictly than pedestrians do.

The movement of traffic tells me when the light changes in my favor. I may pause, but just for a moment, to be sure that no cars are turning in front of me. It is time to step down and walk quickly, using <u>Rule</u>

<u>One</u>. If there are other pedestrians, go with them. There is some safety in numbers. I listen to the cars going my way, and follow the direction they take. This is the time to listen, feel, and think in all directions. Sometimes there is turning traffic for which you must either speed up or slow down. The other side of the street really does exist, and you can get there. By now the last of the cars going your way are passing you on one side, and you are passing the cars waiting on the street you are crossing on the other side of you. Now here is the curb. Sweep it off, step up, and go on your way.

What Goes Through My Mind While Walking Down a Street?

When I was a child I used to hear of people who could dance and talk with their partners at the same time. I thought they had to be very good dancers to do that. When I grew older and learned to dance, I found that it wasn't as hard as I thought it would be. When a blind person walks down a sidewalk, swinging a long white cane, some of the same physical and mental coordination is going on. When walking with a cane you coordinate your own speed and rhythm with your surroundings. There are lots of things you anticipate, notice, and then pass by. Come along as I take a six-block walk through a downtown area.

As I get off the bus, I let the cane tell me if I am in the street or on the curb. It's a deep step to the street. The first swing of the cane finds the curb. The rest of the swing clears the curb, and I step up and go in about two more steps. Now I am at the sidewalk. Along this street there are sections of grassy tree lawn, so I have to keep back from the curb about this distance.

I turn right and get Rule One going. There's traffic in the street on the right, and I'll try to stay an even distance from it. It sounds like people standing and talking near the edge of the walk, so I need to curve around them. Now there's grass on the right, so I let the cane touch it on each swing to that side. The grass won't last long, but it's a good shoreline while it's there.

Some lady in high heels is trying to trot past me. I must not be going fast enough for her. So what! I walk faster than some people and more slowly than others. I'll follow those heels to the end of the block.

I must be nearing the end of the block. I can hear cars crossing in front of me. I should go clear out to the curb on this block. I have turned to go around the corner too soon on other trips here and found myself where I didn't want to be and wasn't sure where I was. At a time like that I try to reverse my course and get back to a known location.

There's the corner with its wheel chair ramp. I back up a step, turn left, and get <u>Rule One</u> going again. There's no good shoreline on this side of the walk. On the return trip there's a good shoreline, a nice cement curb along the inner edge of the walk. Sometimes I drift over and take that side of the walk, anyway. This time I listen.

hard to the traffic on the right and keep it just so far from me. "Oh drat!" I got too close, and the tree is trying to brush my hair for me. People are approaching from ahead, so I narrow the swing of the cane on the left a bit.

There's traffic crossing in front of me, again. I need to notice how long it keeps moving since this time I must cross the street. "Five seconds—ten seconds." No, it changed. Now the cars are going my way. Will I have time to get there before the green light goes stale? "Ten seconds—fifteen—twenty." No, too late. Lights change every thirty seconds in this part of town, so I would rather wait for a fresh start. I'm not perfectly accurate on counting seconds, but I'm close enough to give myself a good idea of when to expect the lights to change. The light changes; no cars turning; I walk; and, what do you know, right up the ramp on the other side.

The next block has a wide sidewalk with tall buildings on the left. There is something going on at the lower edge of my awareness, and I don't think of it most of the time. Background noise reflects off this continuous wall of buildings, and "hearing that wall" makes it easier for me to keep a steady distance from it. These next four blocks have the same feature, but the only time I think of it is in the last block when an alley makes a break in the wall. The cane keeps swinging, according to <u>Rule One</u>, but that is almost as unconscious an act as moving my feet.

Both street and pedestrian traffic are heavier here. There is a person calling out at the far end of the block. Drawing nearer I can tell it is a woman selling fruit. I give her a little more space on the right. There is plenty of traffic to mark the intersection. Just as I come even with the fruit woman, there is a shift in the surrounding noise, and I have passed the buildings. Now which direction was the light green? I wasn't paying enough attention to that. There are cars crossing in front of me, so I'll just walk slowly up to the curb. There are plenty of cars and people to define the red and green light.

Here's the green light, and all the pedestrians are going, which means that no cars are turning. It's a wide street, and I go at a quick pace. At other times I have found a sign post half way across at the edge of the crosswalk, but if I keep to the right I should avoid it.

Mentally I balance all the values. Don't get too close to the cars on the right; avoid the sign on the left; don't trip the pedestrians with the cane; here's the hump in the middle of the street; it's downhill from here; a car is turning the corner in front of me; I pause—it's bigger than I am; and now, the curb, at last. Sweep off the curb, and— whoops! Don't step up here. There are several signposts in the way. Turn toward the corner with one tap of the cane in the street and one tap on the curb. Now the curb is clear, so step up, and just in time. Listen a moment to people and cars for a directional guide, and off we go again.

This block is rather uneventful, and here's the next intersection. There is plenty of traffic, so I know when the light's changing, and there it goes, just in time for me. It isn't quite a straight crossing, but half a step to the right is enough of a correction. I dodge left around the popcorn stand which shows itself in three ways. It blocks the sound of the cars behind it, a sound shadow; the vendor and customers are talking; and you can guess what the last clue is.

Now, for the last two blocks, and this one is plain vanilla. The light changes in my favor just as I pass the last building. "One thousand, two thousand, three thousand." There's the corner, and no cars turning. I still have time to make it.

The crossing is OK, and my building is almost at the end of the block. There's the alley which is about two-thirds of the way. It's time to cross over to the left side of the walk and tap the front of buildings with each swing of the cane.

What I want is a wide entrance with a foot-thick, metal-covered pole at the edge of the walk, but all the buildings here are even with the walk.

Here's a building, more building, a glass door, but it's not set back, more building ... "Bother!" There's the corner, so I passed it. Turn around and go back. There's the building; glass door, more building. Here are the setback and the pole, my building at last. Now it's just two steps and turn right for the swinging door.

Every trip is a bit different, even though some component parts are similar. Just disassemble the parts and shake them up before selecting the items for your next trip. If you keep your landmarks in mind, use your basic techniques, and pay attention to things around you; you'll get there.

Walking with Someone Else

The first thing to remember when you are walking with someone else is that you are still responsible for your own safety. The

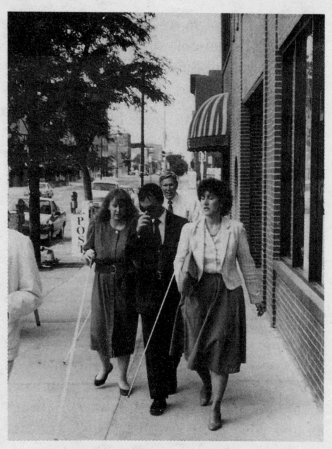

Taking a sighted person's arm does not mean that you can forget to use the cane.

two times I suffered serious injury while walking were while I was with someone else. I falsely and foolishly gave over direction to the sighted person I thought was guiding me. In each case the other person considered that I was managing at least part of my own guidance. The other person may choose the main route, guide you around obstacles, let you know at step-ups and drop-offs, but it is essential for you to pay attention, too.

When I walk with another person, sighted or blind, I find it easier to stay with them if one of us takes the arm of the other. Not everyone likes that physical contact, so I have to divide my attention between where I am going and where the other person is. We can stay close enough for conversation, but the proximity is not as steady.

If you are with a stranger, or even a friend, it is polite to ask, "May I take your arm?" If the other person agrees to your request, take the arm lightly or put your hand on a shoulder. Fall in step. Regardless of whether your companion is sighted or blind, continue using <u>Rule One</u>.

Some of my sighted friends and family members are used to guiding me, and I am confident of their judgment about speed, space, and obstacles. Sometimes I walk directly behind if the space is narrow. When the space opens up, I step up beside them. I do not always judge well where the other people's feet are and step on their shoes. I try to judge their step by the sway of their bodies, but I don't always get it right.

Many guides, such as the people you meet at street corners who offer to help you across the street, are not familiar with how to guide. I may just muddle through, or I may take the time to say something like this: "It is easier if I take your arm. That way, you will be half a step in front, and I can anticipate my step by noticing what you do."

There are circumstances when I make good or bad compromises with the rules. With a guide I sometimes walk along with the cane diagonally across my body while making regular or occasional taps.

Walking Without a Cane

We all walk without a cane sometimes, so let's talk about it. I remember the rule I read in a book about mountain climbing which said that you should always use a rope, but you should climb as if you did not have a rope.

When you are not using a cane, everything else in the environment becomes more important. Whatever you can find with any other sense organ must be evaluated as quickly as possible. In my own home, I try to keep doors open or closed all the way. I swing an arm through a doorway as I near it, just to be sure I am passing through it neatly. Sometimes I touch furniture as I go by. I pause at the top and bottom of stairs, and reach with my foot to locate the first step. When looking for a doorknob or light switch, I make more of a sweeping motion than a straight reach. I sometimes keep my arm across in front of my waist.

One thing I do not do is to hold my arms straight out with the palms forward in the traditional sleep-walker's pose. If I were that uncertain, I would use my cane. The cane looks better and is far more effective.

I walk more slowly without a cane. I do not use a cane within my own home, and rarely enough around my yard. But that is the boundary. Once in a while I will walk a short way around my neighborhood without a cane. And one time, because of freak circumstances, I was caught at night, five blocks from home, on the far side of a traffic circle without a cane. I walked very carefully and a little slower than usual, and made it, but I would not do it if there were another way.

Using a cane is a habit with me, and when I go out, I grab my cane on the way.

■ PUBLIC TRANSPORTATION

Riding Buses and Streetcars

Most trips involve walking at the beginning and end, or even in the middle, so that many skills are used. You need to have the route, destination, and length of the trip in mind before you start. While planning your trip, learn the name and/or number of the bus you want. Buses for different routes may use the same or nearby stops, and you will need to ask before boarding.

You need to know where the stop is: at the corner or around the corner, back from the corner or across the intersection. All of these locations and more are possibilities. In my boyhood and youth I rode streetcars that ran in the center lane of the street. We boarded from an island, sometimes raised and sometimes painted on the street. I had to locate the island by listening to where cars did not run.

With practice you will learn how fast people shuffle along as they step up, pay their fare, get a transfer, and find a seat. Do you need to ask the driver to call your stop for you? The time of boarding is a good time to ask for that help. Sometimes it is wise to confirm your destination with the driver as you near it, especially if it is a long trip. When you get off, remember all those possible locations of the bus stop we mentioned at the beginning of the trip. In unfamiliar areas, I ask where the stop will be for the return trip.

Over the years I have made many mistakes such as waiting at the wrong stop, getting on the wrong bus, getting off too soon or too late, and more. I have paid for these mistakes in time and confusion, but I have learned from them.

Next I will present a step-by-step account of a trip I take frequently. I do this to share what I find necessary and helpful when riding the bus. This trip takes me from work to home.

I go out the door of the building where I work and turn left. At the end of the block there is an oblique left where I again go to the end of the block.

There are three streets that almost come together here to form a series of individual intersections. There are curb cuts for wheelchairs, and if I use them and walk straight, I hit the ramp on the opposite side. At this time of day there is plenty of traffic waiting to go the same way I do. I go when they go, stay parallel to the line of cars on the left, keep between them and the cars waiting their turn on my right. If I step up on grass, I am too far to the right, so I correct to the left. It is about seventy feet to the next corner, and about half of that distance is taken by the entrance to a gas station. I can tell when I am crossing their slanted driveway if one foot is high and one foot is low.

I wait through the cycle of lights and cross the next street. On the curb I walk in two or three steps and turn right. The bus stop is a bus length down, just beyond a plot of dirt with a tree and a trash can. There are often other people waiting for the bus.

There are three routes that use this stop, and two of them will take me where I need to go. Some of the drivers have learned to announce their route as they open the door, so I don't always have to ask. Often there are people getting off, so I wait my turn to board. I step up, put the fare in the box, ask for my kind of transfer to go across a zone line, and find a seat.

Here I digress for a point of philosophy. Drivers and other passengers may encourage you or force you to sit in the "priority seating" at the front of the bus. The choice is still yours to take it or not. I sometimes sit in front and sometimes farther back.

How do I know where to get off? This leg of the trip is short enough so I have learned the pattern of the eight stops. Even if we miss one, and at that time of day we usually hit them all, I can account for the distance. It goes like this: long, medium,

medium, long, very short, long, medium but often missed, medium. After six I get up, approach the driver and ask. I actually count stops on my fingers, but please don't tell my third grade teacher!

The stop where I get off is near the corner, so I walk the few feet and check for the direction of traffic. Sometimes I cross with that noisy bus beside me, but I feel safe because no traffic is coming through that bus. The stop for the next bus is just to the right where I have to thread my way between a trash can, a telephone stand, and a newspaper vending machine, all good landmarks.

For this bus and the next my only fare is my transfer. We go through a distinctive set of turns and up a long hill, but I don't have to notice while going home because I ride to the end of the line.

At this terminal, I walk straight away from the bus, then turn to follow the sidewalk beside the turn-around used by several of the buses. I dodge people, benches, and supporting pillars, and turn out at the second exit, which puts me right at the fire plug beside my bus stop. This time I can only take one of the three buses that stop here, and sometimes they line up, so I may have to back up fifty feet for mine. I have made a few "bus stop" acquaintances who sometimes give me the word.

This leg of the trip takes about twenty minutes. We start off around the terminal and, after a quarter of a mile, in, around, and out of a traffic circle. Those turns are distinctive. We go about four miles with very few people getting on or off. Then we come to a major intersection for which we must wait through at least one cycle of the lights and with the stop after we cross. After the next stop, which we do not always make, the bus makes an oblique left turn, and I sigh with anticipation because it is my last landmark. I get up when the bus shifts into high gear. At my stop I go back across the street we just crossed and walk two short blocks to my home.

I know that this description is long, but it is the "one bite at a time" approach to eating an elephant. No two trips are exactly the same, but you may find some of these techniques useful as you develop your own.

Subways, Escalators, and Elevators

The first thing people want to know about subways is the location of the platform edge. I slide my cane tip along to locate the edge, step back from it, and respect it. As I walk along subway platforms, I walk a little more slowly than usual, and I swing my cane a little wider than usual. I also slide the cane on the surface, the only time I use this otherwise poor technique. I want to know immediately if the cane drops over the edge. I expect people to criticize me about this point, so go ahead. The one thing I do not do is step sideways. The cane has been ahead of me, not to the side.

When the train comes, and after the door opens, put the cane tip on the floor of the

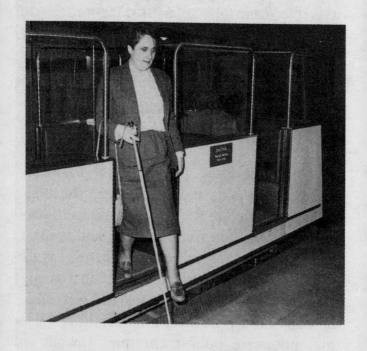

*Light rail transportation causes
no problems to a good cane user.*

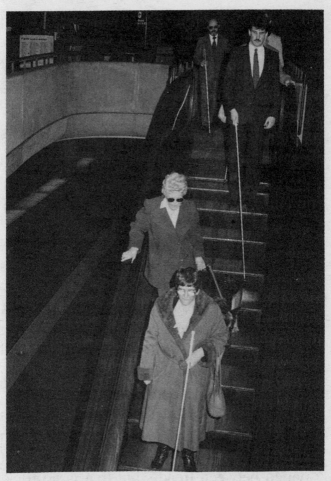

*Escalators are no problem either
with proper cane technique.*

car before you step in just to be sure you are not trying to enter the gap between cars. When you get off, let the cane tip go first to be sure that there is a platform waiting for you.

Are there stairs, escalators or elevators to take you up and down? Stairs have been discussed earlier. For escalators, I only know one warning and two tricks, and they are not exclusive to blind people. The warning is that an escalator is a powerful, moving machine. Cooperate with it as it helps you, and you will get there. Use the hand-rail, and don't play around. The first trick is, if I am not sure if an escalator is going up or down, I pause in front of it and feel the hand-rail. The other trick is one of balance as I step on or off a moving platform. When I step on, and I feel the stair treads dividing under my feet, I step up or down so that my whole foot is on one tread, not divided between treads, but that is no trick. It is just common sense.

Treat elevators with the same respect you treat the platform edge. Let the cane tell you that there is something solid ahead of you to step on. This is no time to enact bad elevator jokes.

Airports, Train and Bus Stations

Transportation terminals tend to have several features in common. There are long distances to cover and large open areas with arrangements of furniture in the middle. The ticket counter is relatively close to the entrance, relative to the size of the terminal, that is.

The next part of the trip may cover several hundred yards of corridors including an array of modern miracle transportation: moving sidewalks, people movers, monorails and more. Little children think they are fun; I must be getting old. At the end of this part of the trip you must find just the right door and play the ticket game again.

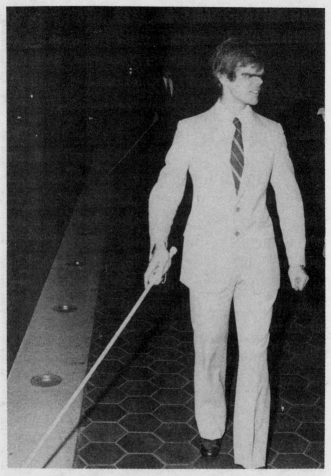

Maintaining contact with the platform edge is a good way of traveling safely in a metro station.

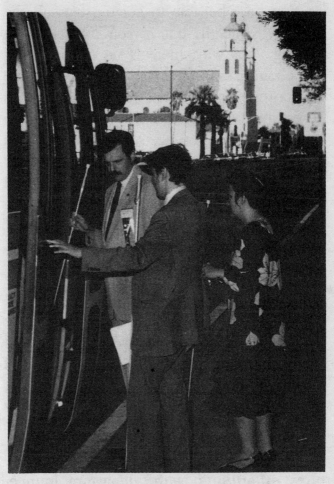

They won't miss the bus.

You may be able to get most or all the way by yourself, but if you need help in finding your way, there is no use in being shy about asking for help. A personal guide may range from necessary to helpful to bothersome. As hard as it sometimes is to find help when you need it, sometimes it is harder to get rid of help when you don't want it any more. Some trips are once and never again, and I need more help then. Some trips are regulars, and I need little if any help then.

The job of the blind traveler is to learn and keep in mind the gate number and departure time. The guide, then, needs only to locate and steer, not to investigate and govern. Guides may try to investigate and govern, anyway, but it is your trip, not theirs. You make the decisions, so you stay in control.

In my experience, one of the distinct features of airports is the departure lounge. That is where you may have your ticket taken away from you, be pre-boarded, be helped at the right or wrong time with the right or wrong amount of help.

I have found it informative to hear what airline personnel say to each other about me: "Should we take his ticket?" That was when I clutched my ticket and gently found a seat to wait in. It was not the same seat I had before I went up to ask my question, but I still had my ticket and boarded when I chose.

There was the time when three flights were called before mine. Everyone walked around the edge of the lounge, avoiding the central area. I decided that benches or plants must be blocking that area. I could hear where tickets were being taken. When my flight was called, I took the "round" trip and found the departure gate myself. That was when I heard, "He didn't ask for any help." I don't always insist on being that independent, but that day I did.

Train stations may or may not be as big as airports, but they share the same obstacles. Trains are long, so platforms have to be long. Some train platforms are raised above the level of the tracks, so remember the rules from the subway lesson. Locate the platform edge, and respect it. Do not step sideways. Let your cane tell you that there is something solid to step on: up, down, and level.

Bus stations range in size from a driveway beside a small-town drug store to a city block or more. In bus stations, you need to get to the right boarding gate, and there is often a loud noise when you get there. Sometimes the distance from the boarding gate to the bus door is short and obvious, and you can find it easily. Sometimes the bus you want is behind or beyond three others, all of which are roaring along with their engines on "high idle". If you know where to go, then go ahead. Remember <u>Rule One</u>. If you don't know where to go, ask for help. All that noise to a blind person masks other useful sounds. The equivalent situation to a sighted person would be turning out the lights or flooding the area with fog.

■ TIMES AND PLACES WITHOUT THE USUAL LANDMARKS

Grocery Stores

If I am going alone, and I know what I want and where it is, I find movement easiest with my cane in front while holding the front end of the grocery cart and pulling it behind me. It steers better that way. If I am shopping with another person, I find that store aisles are too narrow for two people and a cart. That is when I follow my guide with my hand on a shoulder. The cart needs to go at the front or the back of the procession, a matter of personal choice.

Most of the time I am an organized shopper, preparing my grocery list beforehand. If I know the layout of the store, I think of each section and decide what to buy as I mentally walk around. If the store is new to me, and all stores are new the first time, I do some preparation, anyway. The more I am going to buy, the more help I need, so

I ask the store for one of their staff to help in my selections. You have to be specific when designating items: tuna, oil-packed or water-packed; cereal, which size; bananas, how green. Finding a time that is good for you to shop and the store to help is a matter of juggling schedules.

In years past, I used a two-wheeled fold-up cart for pulling my groceries home. The cart had a bad habit of getting too close and running over my heel. In order to keep the cart in its place behind me, I held my arm straight down and against my side. That position kept the wheels back from me.

How Do You Walk in Ice, Snow, and Rain?

Ice, snow, and rain have this in common: they make the footing slippery. How do I keep from giving a skating demonstration and falling on my dignity? I walk a little more slowly, keep my knees slightly bent, and take shorter steps. I also put my feet down flat, not striding out with the heel landing first. I may not move fast, but I do move and stay upright.

If the snow is light or fresh, I dig my cane through it, and with the combination of sound and touch I can tell what is there. If the snow is too deep to dig through or it is packed and frozen, the cane must find something above the surface to identify as a landmark. Sometimes packed snow on the sidewalk and loose snow beside it show enough difference to help. Taller landmarks are helpful, such as bushes, fences, sign posts, and parked cars. Snow covers many of the usual landmarks, but it can become a landmark, itself. One winter it stayed so cold for so long that I used a particular snow bank as a landmark on the way to a friend's house.

When the snow is deep and soft, it weighs down branches which hang in front of you. One advantage of a long cane is that you can reach up and tap a branch so it will release its burden of snow before you walk under it. Well, it works sometimes.

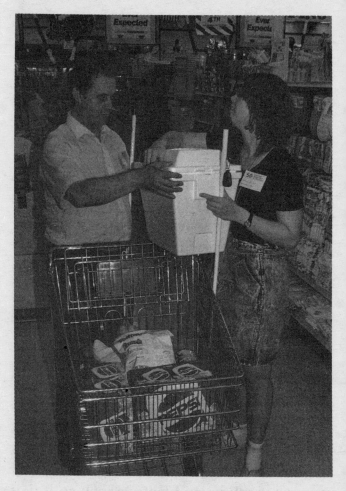

Not by bread alone. . .
It also requires to and from the store.

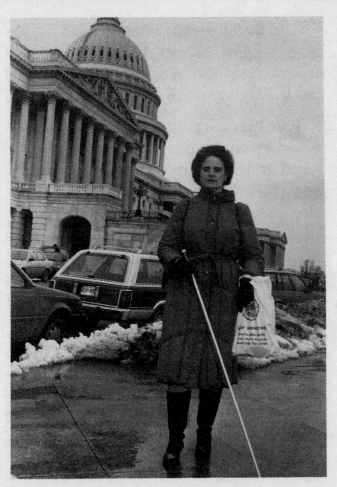

Neither rain nor snow. . .
She walks to the Capitol to talk
with members of Congress about
matters affecting the blind.

The world sounds different with a covering of snow. Echoes disappear. Distances expand. I navigate more by dead reckoning and less by my usual landmarks.

Rain may not change the footing as much as snow and ice do, but it can change the sound of things in its own way. Cars hissing by on wet streets mask other sounds. Rustling raincoats do the same. Hats, scarves and hoods all influence what you hear in different ways, and you may want to think of that along with the weather. I am rarely out in rain so hard that it covers all other sounds.

It may take longer to get places in the rain. I often listen harder and wait longer to know where things are and when things happen. Here is another practical use for the long cane: finding the depth and width of curbside puddles.

How About Suburban and Rural Roads with No Sidewalks?

I like to get routes, distances, and landmarks well in mind before starting. There is more area in which to get lost, and fewer people from whom to ask directions. I take my longest cane and swing it rather widely. I move along at a good clip because there are greater distances to cover. I still have to stay alert for traffic on the road, as well as mailboxes and ditches beside it.

I usually stay on the shoulder of the roadway, but sometimes I take short excursions to explore for a sidewalk which may appear for a while, or a front walk, driveway, or other landmark that would help me keep track of what is about and around. I like to stay close to the road, because that is the main landmark. The direction of the sun, wind, and distant sounds can also be used as a guide and landmark.

Are There Roads and Intersections Unsafe for Any Pedestrian?

I am one of those people who finds the "wet paint" sign and wonders if the paint is still wet. That same rebellious, disbelieving streak comes out when people tell me not to attempt certain streets or intersections because they are too dangerous or complicated for me. I always wonder if they mean "because I am blind."

I usually learn something about these places before testing them for myself. Is there another street or intersection a block or two from there that would get me to my destination just as well? The answer is sometimes "yes" and sometimes "no." I know some "nervous nay-sayers" who simply have no faith in the travel abilities of blind people. I also know some "supporting stalwarts" who recognize realistic obstacles.

When it comes time for me to make my own decision, I take it slowly, allowing plenty of time on my schedule. I also pick an off-peak time for traffic. There is no doubt about it, I have made mistakes! Once I found that the roadway dropped immediately into a 3-foot wide ditch at the bottom of a 50-degree hill. The cars going by fanned me with their breeze. I never went back there. Another time I walked over an area of hedges, potted plants, no proper sidewalks, becoming somewhat disoriented before coming to the other side. I was glad I had only gone through the confusing part of that one, and not the dangerous part.

Sometimes I have had satisfying success. I have stood at an intersection for many minutes, listening to the traffic to learn where the movement went, and when the directions changed. Then I decided I could make it, and did. To another blind person, I would say, "Gather all your skills and use your best judgment for evaluating the situation before and during the trip. If necessary, be willing to find another route for the next time."

Picnics, Hiking, and
Rough Country

Do you go for picnics or hikes in the country? When I go on these trips, I take my sturdiest cane along. It is just as important here as anywhere else to use the cane and to keep track of landmarks and directions. When I arrive at a new area, I do as many people do; I try to get an idea of what is around me. Are there buildings, roads, rocks, trees, or open areas? Is there a slope to the land, and what is the direction of the sun, wind, and noises? I may do some short-range exploring while keeping track of my point of reference, be it a car or a picnic table.

Since I am the only man in my family and the strongest one of us, I get to carry the picnic cooler from the car to the table, but I still use my cane. The cane is held somehow or other in front, whether I am being guided or carrying this two-handed burden alone. My shins want the cane to tell them when we arrive at the bench.

When hiking beside someone else, I still protect myself with the cane. Some trails are well-worn and obvious to the feet, so I may walk alone and use <u>Rule One</u>, the side-to-side swing of the cane. On some narrow trails I let my guide take one end of the cane while I hold the other end. Since I am without the cane as a bumper, I work out signals with my partner such as "left around the rock," or "up and over the log." I try to get my partner to put the functional word first and not at the end of a long, descriptive sentence. By the time I listen to "There's a bend in the trail up here with a tree on one side and a cliff on the other, so I guess you'd better stay to the right," I may already have met my fate.

When it comes to clambering over hills and boulders, some of the cane technique gets rather informal. I still use the cane to locate the next place my foot is going. Sometimes there is as much poking and probing as swinging the cane from side to side. I rarely jump, and only when I am very sure of where I will land. When the rocks and hills get very steep, it may be more practical to slip the cane under my belt or abandon it altogether, and just use hands and feet.

If you want to use a directional compass, you need to have a good idea of where you are going before you begin. You must make the compass work for you along with the other tools you use. Keep a record of landmarks, distances, and compass bearings. If you are going very far, you need more instruction in orienteering than I can give you here.

When I am entangled in bushes and trees with interlocking branches as high as my head, I am usually in someone's back yard or in a city park. Only a few times have I been in rough country where this condition lasted. If the usual city technique of swinging the cane along the ground is just not telling you enough, and the branches are getting in your face, try this.

Bring the cane up at a diagonal in front of your body, across at head level, and down at a diagonal to the other side. For the next step, reverse the direction. The path of the cane is an X with a loop at the top. I go rather slowly when I do this, and I am usually holding back branches with my free hand. This really is a "wild woods" technique. Do not use it around people or other works of the human race such as windows. In all the years of travel I have behind me, my total use of this technique probably does not exceed ten minutes.

■ CARE AND FEEDING OF THE LONG WHITE CANE

Wash, Feed, and Dress Your Cane

The washing part is obvious, but I am a poor one to tell you, since I don't do it often enough, myself. Collapsible canes that are held together by an internal elastic cord need watching. Keep track of the wear on the elastic cord, and be smart enough to replace it the day before it breaks. Of course, it is better to be a month early than a day late.

Cane tips last me anywhere from a few weeks to a few months. I carry a spare tip with me most of the time. A cane tip with a hole in it sounds different from a tip without the hole, and that is the sign to carry a spare tip all the time. I have worn out or lost tips unexpectedly. The unprotected end of any cane, especially fiberglass, is damaged quickly when rubbed against concrete. Just wave the cane, and keep the tapping to a minimum.

Does your cane have reflective tape on it? If not, you could put some on it anywhere along the stem. It is an investment in night-time safety. Reflective surfaces need to be kept clean or replaced to maintain their reflective value.

If you associate with other blind people, as I do, you may want some unique mark on your cane. I write my name in Braille on Dymo tape and stick it on the bottom end of the handle.

Where Does the Cane Go When Not in Use?

When answering this question, you discover the great advantage of the folding or collapsible cane. Those styles can fit in a pocket, purse, on a lap, or under a chair very easily.

There are two horizontal dimensions and one vertical dimension. Find some place out of the way: lying on the floor under a chair or table, standing in a corner, or leaning against a wall. Be sure that the cane is lying flat on the floor and not resting on something that holds it an inch or two above the floor where it will be just high enough to trip the unsuspecting passer-by. In some crowded areas "up" is the only way left. When I am seated, I sometimes lean the cane from the floor to my shoulder, hooked behind my heel.

Once in a restaurant, I lost the tip while retrieving the cane from a tiny place behind the booth. I remember that incident, and sometimes I take the tip off before jamming the cane into tight places. In air travel I stick the cane in some out-of-the-way place but do not let the crew take it away from me. The regulations are now on <u>our</u> side.

Which Hand Do You Cane With?

The most obvious answer to this question is that you cane with your dominant hand. I am right-handed, but I trade off when I carry a heavy object. There may be a landmark I want to check on the other side. When I am walking with someone else, holding on or not, it may be better to have the cane on the other side to stay away from feet or another cane. If someone is holding my cane arm, it restricts the movement. I don't want that. I have had enough practice with my left hand so that I am fully adequate, but I am still more comfortable with the cane in the right hand. The question of which hand you use is a matter of the convenience of the moment.

■ THOUGHTS AND EXPERIENCES ON CANE TRAVEL

How Long Does It Take to Learn Cane Travel?

In order to answer this question, you must consider three major variable factors: 1. your background; 2. your aptitude; and 3. the amount of time available.

I will give some numbers from my experience, but not until I expand on these factors.

Background: Are you familiar with the area where you will be traveling? Do you know where some of the streets and buildings are? Are you used to the roar of the city, the hush of the suburbs, the quiet of the country? Do you know that streets have names and numbers, and that buildings have numbers, but sometimes have names? Do you start off fearful of traffic, or just unfamiliar with it? Are you familiar with traffic and the way it moves so that you know what to expect of it?

Aptitude: Are you used to finding your own way, or have people always taken you places and told you when to stop and go? Let me recall two extremes of aptitude.

The youth was newly blind and in his late teens. He came from a rural setting where he had often gone on cross-country treks when he was sighted. There was a touch of youthful rebellion in him. It seemed as though his needs would be met by handing him a cane, reading him <u>Rule One</u>, and getting out of his way. He did go through several lessons, but he never needed to repeat them for practice. He was a natural traveler.

The lady was newly blind and middle-aged. She was from an urban setting, but was not used to getting places alone. She was very comfortable with her friends in her living room. During lessons she made the narrowest possible interpretation of instructions and then paused to ask, "Is this right?" I could not bring her to the recognition of her own responsibility to judge each situation. We parted company disappointed with each other.

There are people who would associate some of these characteristics with being sighted or blind, but I have met people in both groups with odd mixtures of these characteristics.

The amount of time available: Time should be measured in two ways: the number of hours per day and week, and the number of months to be filled with this schedule. When I began as a student in a residential orientation center, I was spending fifteen to twenty hours a week in guided practice. It worked well for me. I have known people who made good progress with four to five hours of guided practice in a week. It seems to me that anything under three hours in a week would be getting rather thin. These hours I am talking about are hours spent on specific skill practice. They cannot be the only time spent using the cane. After all, you are learning these skills to use them in everyday life, so <u>every</u> time you go out, take your cane and use what you have been learning. As with any skill, the more you use it, the faster you will improve.

The next time you send a letter, grab your cane and walk down to the corner mailbox. Find excuses to take short trips here and there. There must be some places you want to go, so walk there with your cane. Take the cane <u>every</u> time you go out. It is this kind of constant purposeful practice that locks in the lessons and speeds the learning process. If the only time you use your cane is during the three hours a week you have lessons, and every other time you go somewhere it is on the arm of your guide, you are not going to learn how to travel alone.

One thing that helped me a great deal was being with other blind people who took short trips together. We walked within the buildings, around the grounds, and out for snacks. There is nothing like peer pressure, seeing that they can do it and having them expect you to join them. Aren't you just as smart as they are? And if you are still a beginner, you don't have to be in front.

I spent an intensive six weeks on travel and reached a satisfactory level of skill. Most people I know who worked steadily for several hours a week, plus out-of-class "just walking around" became good travelers or made as much progress as they were going to make for a good foundation in travel in two to three months. That is from starting as a beginner.

Can a Blind Person Teach Cane Travel?

By the time I tried teaching other people, I was a good traveler. Wherever I lived, I had to learn the area, but there was little difference in difficulty from one place to the next. I crossed narrow and wide streets with straight or angled crossings. There were traffic islands and multiple-phase traffic lights with more or less traffic. I had to think about some intersections more than others, but I went where I wanted to go.

When I planned lessons for beginning students, I had to consider the difficulties of the lesson for each day and gradually increase the level of challenge. That was my first surprise as a teacher. I scouted the area of each lesson to identify landmarks, challenges, and hazards. Having given route instructions at the beginning of the walk, I then preceded or followed the student. There were always certain places where I wanted to be nearby to evaluate how the student met the challenge of the day. The difficulty for any teacher is knowing when to let the student work out the problem alone, and when to step in with further instruction. What we did was very basic. At first you walk up and down the block, then around the block. You cross narrow, quiet streets, and then busier streets with traffic lights. You work on short routes the student wants to accomplish, then longer trips. Some lessons are just for practice, but later they are more and more to meet the student's needs. You work indoors, outdoors, and take buses. After a while, you don't have to repeat lessons for practice. Just be sure that the instructions are understood, and send them on their way. My teacher ended the course by working us through a 3-1/2 mile hike around a section of the city. It gave us students a true sense of accomplishment to be able to manage that trip and what it had to offer. This seems like the time for the teacher to say, "You don't need me any more. Congratulations, and goodbye."

No One Has to Do Everything Perfectly

One of the things we all need to do is to find a doorway as we walk beside a wall. Many of us slide the cane along at the angle of the floor and wall until the cane hits the door frame. That method works, but I want to point out its weaknesses. Traffic patterns put us on the right side of the path; the wall is often on our right; and most of us are right-handed. All that means that we are not covering the body with the cane, thus leaving us open to a collision. I shift the cane to the hand opposite the wall to give myself at least some coverage, in case there is something or someone in the way. Of course, <u>Rule One</u> says I should continue tapping the cane from side to side to clear the space in front of me, but with my stride of two-and-a-half feet I will only touch the wall every five feet and miss a narrow door. Sometimes I swing the cane in the hand away from the wall and slide the near hand lightly along the wall. This last method may be the best compromise.

When I lose track of where I am when I am walking around, and I find someone of whom I can ask directions, my first question is, "What's the name of this street?" I may know enough to find my own way with that information. If I have not learned enough, I ask, "How do I get to ...?" If I have to ask another person later, I ask.

I am a poor judge of the distance ahead of my cane. I tend to tap ankles and trip people. If I want to be sure, I have to give myself far more space than I really need. It is even worse if the person ahead is using a cane, and I hear the tap which is five feet ahead of where they are.

When I am walking directly behind a guide as we pass through a narrow space, I often step on the heels of my guide. I know you are supposed to be able to tell which foot is forward by the swing of the shoulders, but I don't always coordinate well. I have to take very short steps to keep from stepping on them. It keeps me out of step, but it also keeps my feet off of theirs.

I often have the bad habit of letting my head nod forward. Didn't we all have mothers who said: "Keep your head up. Stand up straight!" The practical reason for keeping my head up is to avoid using it as a bumper. The cane is supposed to be the bumper. It is supposed to be in front all the time. Better the cane should get scars, not the body.

There are some days I always drift to the right and other days I drift to the left. If paying more attention to the line of traffic or to the shoreline doesn't help, I bring my cane hand back to the middle of my body and concentrate on keeping the swing of the cane even from side to side. "Back to basics" straightens me out.

The first trip to almost any place usually includes lots of exploration and false starts. Sometimes that continues for several trips until I learn the local geography. If you can learn faster than I can, more power to you.

There is one situation when I learned to look lost on purpose. It is a crowded theater lobby during intermission when I am trying to find the men's room. I take a few steps this way and that way, then pause and look around with a confused expression on my face. Pretty soon someone will offer help, at which point I suddenly regain all my travel skills.

What About Other Travel Aids, Dogs, and Electronics?

I tend to be a practical person. The rule is: "If it works for you, use it." I was introduced first to the cane and was fortunate in that I had a good teacher. I learned to travel independently, and it has served me very well.

There are blind people who travel well with a cane and those who travel poorly with a cane. There are blind people who travel well with a guide dog and those who travel poorly with a guide dog. I will tell you what I know about dogs.

Any reputable guide dog school insists on giving travel training along with the dog, and that is an advantage. Canes do not come with training attached. A dog can offer companionship. A dog has some memory of its own and may help in confusing or dangerous situations. Dogs also make mistakes, just like their masters. There is truth in all of these points. I like other people's dogs, but I do not want the responsibilities of feeding, grooming, curbing, and health care that go with owning a dog. If it is right for you, do it. I think it is more important that you get places conveniently and safely than how you get there. It is the human that makes the difference, not the cane or the dog.

Over the past several decades, I have heard of electronic travel aids that were attached to the cane, attached to the forehead, or held in the hand. Each one gave off its own sound or vibration. Each one had advantages: locating objects at a distance without touching them, locating obstacles above cane level, being less "obvious"—not always an advantage. They have come, and they have gone, and the cane and the dog remain. I do not mean to say that there will never be an electronic travel device that lasts, but it seems to be over the horizon. The cane and the dog have been here for many years and are still here.

SONGS

THE WHITE CANE FREEDOM MARCH

by Thomas Bickford, Debbie Brown, Lloyd Rasmussen and Ken Silberman

To the Tune of: "As Those Caissons Go Rolling Along"

Over hill, over dale, we will hit the
  concrete trail;
As our white canes go tapping along.
Down the block, cross the street, walking
  on our own two feet;
As our white canes go tapping along.
On the job or at home, wherever we may
  roam,
Yes, independent and free! NFB!
We can find our way at night or in
  the day;
As our white canes go tapping along.

On a bus, on a train, even flying
  on a plane;
As our white canes go tapping along.
As we board, find our seat, no great
  danger shall we meet;
As our white canes go tapping along.
We're the able blind, so leave your
  carts behind.
Don't put us in your holding tanks!
  No thanks!
We'll meet no harm. Take back your
  helping arm.
As our white canes go tapping along.

On we go at full speed. No contraptions
  do we need;
As our white canes go tapping along.
No rough tiles for our feet, nor the
  traffic signal's tweet;
As our white canes go tapping along.
No Ph.D.'s, just skillful travelers, please,
Teaching blind people to be free! NFB!
And the rehab snobs can go and find
  real jobs;
As our white canes go tapping along.

THE LAMENT OF
THE FOLDING CANE

by Thomas Bickford

*To the tune of "A Pretty Girl is
Like a Melody"*

My folding cane was quite reliable
When it was still brand new.
I'd fold it and then swing it again.
I'd make it small, then use it all
The time, no matter when.

My folding cane is just a memory,
Now that it fell apart.
The elastic stretched and broke.
Four short canes are a joke,
And now my one-piece cane's the cane
That has won my heart.

SOURCES
OF CANES

In many cities there are agencies that sell canes, where you may examine them before you buy. If there is a cane mentioned in this booklet that you cannot find locally, you may contact:

Materials Center
National Center for the Blind
1800 Johnson Street
Baltimore, Maryland 21230
Telephone: (410) 659-9314

Catalogs are available in print and Braille. If the National Center for the Blind does not carry the cane in stock, it will either get the cane for you or refer you to a source.

BIBLIOGRAPHY

Benson, Stephen O. "So What About Independent Travel." *The Braille Monitor*, January, 1985, pp 30-40.

Blasch, B. B., Long, R. G., and Griffin, Shirley N. "Results of a National Survey of Electronic Travel Aid Use." *Journal of Visual Impairment and Blindness*, November, 1989, v. 33, n 9, pp 449-453.

Dodds, A. G., and Davis, D. P. "Assessment and Training of Low Vision Clients for Mobility." *Journal of Visual Impairment and Blindness*, November, 1989, v 83, n 9, pp 439-446.

Kruger, Irving J. "Orientation and Mobility in the Vocational Area." *New Outlook for the Blind*, March, 1960, v 54, n 3, pp 87-90.

National Conference on Mobility and Orientation: (Introduction), *New Outlook for the Blind*, March, 1960, v 54, n 3, pp 77-81.

Nichols, Allan. "Why Use the Long White Cane?" *The Braille Monitor*, February, 1992, pp 54-58.

Pogrund, R. L., and Rosen, S. J. "The Preschool Blind Child Can be a Cane User." *Journal of Visual Impairment and Blindness*, November, 1989, v 83, n 9, pp 431-439.

Rusalem, Herbert. "The Dilemma in Training Mobility Instructors." *New Outlook for the Blind*, March, 1960, v 54, n 3, pp 82-87.

Sauerberger, Dona. "Cane Technique: Tricks of the Trade." *Metropolitan Washington Orientation and Mobility Association Newsletter*, March, 1992.

Sauerberger, Dona. "Readers' Comments on Teaching Cane Techniques." *Metropolitan Washington Orientation and Mobility Association Newsletter*, May, 1992, pp 3-4.

Wainapel, S. F. "Attitudes of Visually Impaired Persons Toward Cane Use." *Journal of Visual Impairment and Blindness*, November, 1989, v 83, n 9, pp 446-448.

Whitstock, Robert H. "Orientation and Mobility for Blind Children." *New Outlook for the Blind*, March, 1960, v 54, n 3, pp 90-94.

Willoughby, Doris, and Duffy, Sharon. *Handbook for Itinerant and Resource Teachers of Blind and Visually Impaired Students*. Baltimore: National Federation of the Blind, 1989.

If you or a friend would like to remember the National Federation of the Blind in your will, you can do so by employing the following language:

"I give, devise, and bequeath unto National Federation of the Blind, 1800 Johnson Street, Baltimore, Maryland 21230, a District of Columbia nonprofit corporation, the sum of $ --- (or "--- percent of my net estate" or "The following stocks and bonds: ---") to be used for its worthy purposes on behalf of blind persons."

National Federation of the Blind
You can help us spread the word...

...about our Braille Readers Are Leaders contest for blind schoolchildren, a project which encourages blind children to achieve literacy through Braille.

...about our scholarships for deserving blind college students.

...about Job Opportunities for the Blind, a program that matches capable blind people with employers who need their skills.

...about where to turn for accurate information about blindness and the abilities of the blind.

Most importantly, you can help us by sharing what you've learned about blindness in these pages with your family and friends. If you know anyone who needs assistance with the problems of blindness, please write:

Marc Maurer, President
1800 Johnson Street, Suite 300
Baltimore, Maryland 21230-4998
Your contribution is tax-deductible.